The Bathtub Yoga & Relaxation Book

YOGA IN THE BATH FOR ENERGY, VITALITY & PLEASURE

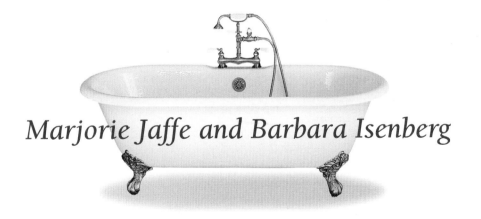

Marjorie Jaffe and Barbara Isenberg

HEALTHY LIVING PUBLICATIONS

Summertown, Tennessee

Cover & interior design: John Wincek
Model photography: Warren Jefferson
Interior photos: © 2000 Corbis Images, Getty Images
Bathtub photos: Sunrise Specialty Co., Berkeley, Cal.

Printed in Hong Kong.

Healthy Living Publications
a division of Book Publishing Company
P.O. Box 99
Summertown, TN 38483
888-260-8458

ISBN 1-57067-128-1

Library of Congress Cataloging-in-Publication Data

Jaffe, Marjorie.
 The bathtub yoga & relaxation book : yoga in the bath for energy, vitality and pleasure / Marjorie Jaffe and Barbara Isenberg.
  p. cm.
 ISBN 1-57067-128-1
 1. Aquatic exercises. 2. Yoga. 3. Baths. 4. Relaxation. I. Title: Bathtub yoga and relaxation book. II. Isenberg, Barbara. III. Title.
 RA781.17 .J345 2002
 613.7'16--dc21

                                        2002004914

09 08 07 06 05 04   2 3 4 5 6 7 8 9

About Sunrise Specialty antique bathtubs

Sunrise Specialty was founded as Sunrise Salvage in Berkeley in 1972. We were a local salvage yard that specialized in Victorian building material. We believe that style is timeless, and it is our love for the old that has allowed us to grow to where we are today. We applaud and support Marjorie and Barbara for creating this book.

Robert E. Mautte, Jr.
Sunrise Specialty Co.

Contents

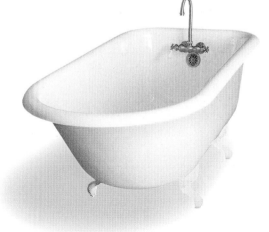

To our readers

We hope that this book will provide serenity and physical comfort during these challenging times.

Acknowledgments

Thanks to our good friends and professional colleagues who helped with our book in immeasurable ways.

- Eleanora Lipton, Registered Polarity Practitioner, Certified Massage Therapist, Intuitive Yoga Instructor, Owner Atlanta Polarity Center, for her careful review of our book and with Alexandra Faer Bryan for their Therapeutic Art of Polarity

- Edwige Gilbert, our beautiful yoga model and yoga expert for her contribution to our book. Deborah DeVoursney and Tal Zadok Kazaz, Yoga Instructors and our models

- Jo Sgammato, certified Integral Yoga Teacher and Mary Leck, Shiatsu Practitioner and Yoga Instructor

- Pat Sarto, Cosmetologist and Renata Floyd, Esthetician

- Sue Zeckendorf, Literary Agent

- John Nowakowski, Chef of the Regency Spa

- Ellen Lieberman, Stylist

We heartily thank our publisher, Bob Holzapfel, and all the great people at Healthy Living Publications. We're grateful to Cynthia Holzapfel, our editor, for her superior knowledge, taste, and heart.

We'd like to thank John Wincek for his outstanding design of the book.

Barbara and Marjorie are grateful for the opportunity to work together again.

Marjorie thanks both her mother and mother-in-law, who always stand by her; her daughter Dr. Bryce, who turned and twisted her beautiful body in the tub to help design some of the exercises; her husband, for his creative contributions; and her son, for his humor and sound advice.

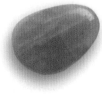

The Bathtub Yoga & Relaxation Book

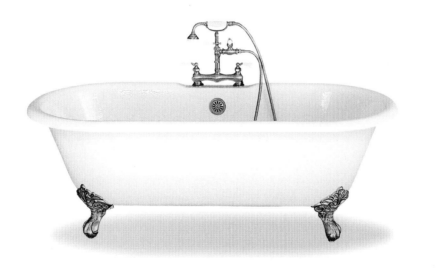

Introduction

The bath is a sanctuary—a peaceful place to relax and let go of tension; a private space to clean away everything on your mind and take time to unwind. Many of us have lost the ability to relax. Our day begins in a rush. We continue the chaotic pace throughout the day and then fit in a whole day's worth of responsibilities from the time we return home until we go to sleep.

A constant state of stress is exhausting and doesn't contribute to a finely tuned body machine. The breathing practices, yoga meditations and positions, and gentle stretches in this book will enhance your bath time and slow your body's rhythm. The more relaxation you experience, the more energy you will have afterwards.

For many, taking a bath is synonymous with stress relief. Warmth and water are two of the best sources for relaxation and comfort to the body. When you sink into the tub, your body releases tension as it stops resisting gravity. The buoyancy of the bathtub water bears your weight and frees your body.

Although we read articles and talk to friends about how to reduce stress, it may be difficult to incorporate a relaxation technique on a regular basis. Getting in the water, however, is joyful. Starting your morning with a bath or looking forward to a pleasant soak in the evening can help get you through the day. Why not combine the everyday experience of bathing with yoga, meditations, and gentle stretching?

Yoga is an ancient practice for increasing flexibility and balance in your body, mind, and spirit. The yoga practices in this book are not meant to be a strenuous workout. We are combining the meditative and calming traditions of both yoga and bathing. The use of scented

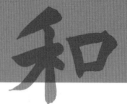

oils, natural lighting, and peaceful sound can fill all your senses and add to the pleasure of bath time. You can create a self-rejuvenation ritual anytime and anywhere there's a tub.

Every culture has its bathing rituals. The practice of hydrotherapy, using bath and water for healing and comfort, has existed since ancient times. Ritual bathing is traceable to early Egypt and Greece. Public baths, "thermaes," with beautiful interiors of rich mosaics, marble, and glazed metals, were developed by the Romans. Japanese soaking tubs have been popular for centuries. And today, jacuzzis and hot tubs are showing up everywhere. Breathing, meditating, and stretching in the bathtub can become a natural ritual for our culture.

Bath time is already sacred to some; others have not yet realized how valuable this time could be. Bath time yoga can become a magical experience; all you feel is the exhilaration, not the work.

Bathe every day and sickness will avoid you. HINDU PROVERB

The Bathtub Yoga and Relaxation Book

There are 3 sections in *The Bathtub Yoga and Relaxation Book:*

Yoga Breathing Practices

pranayama

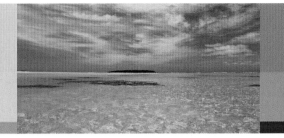

Body Relaxation

water yoga and stretches

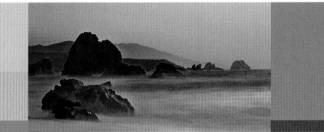

Mind Relaxation

meditations and aromatherapy

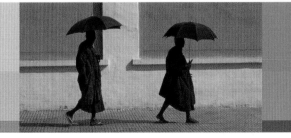

Yoga Breathing Practices

Pranayama

Yoga teaches that as you become aware and focus on your inhalation and exhalation, your mind calms down and relaxes. Many of us already take a bath to relax; adding structured breathing practices will increase your relaxation.

Stress affects the way you breathe. When stress becomes overwhelming, your breathing becomes faster and more shallow. With yoga, you can learn to control the pace and depth of your breathing. The oxygen-rich air you bring into your body adds to your relaxation.

You've been told to "take a deep breath" when you're feeling stress. It doesn't mean to shut down and count to 10. It means to inhale deeply and fill your lungs with fresh air, then exhale and eliminate all the used air. Breathing is both conscious and unconscious, so try to remember to pull air into your lungs as often as you can. Oxygen nourishes all the cells in the body.

There are different ways to practice deep breathing. All of them transport more air into and out of your lungs. When you become truly relaxed, your pulse and heart rate become lower and healthier. You have more energy in your body and your mind. Slow, deep, conscious breathing quiets the mind and creates a serene feeling.

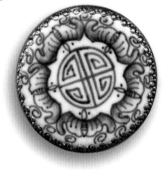

Body Relaxation

Water Yoga and Stretches

Classical yoga postures are called Asanas. We've modified some traditional Asanas so they can be done in the bathtub. Stay focused, aware, and centered in your mind; feel comfort and balance in your body. Let your body sense where all its parts are, and remain aware of your breathing. This is a special time for you, so stay in the present moment.

In the stretching section, you'll be shown certain movements that are similar to what we do instinctively and automatically to feel good. We naturally curl and spread our toes, bend our arms and legs, and roll our neck and shoulders. Other stretches focus on muscle groups which hold tension. All these exercises should feel comfortable; don't believe that if there's no pain, there's no gain. The good news is that stretching your muscles and joints is much easier on your body in warm water.

Stretching is often a neglected aspect of the daily workout. But it is absolutely necessary to keep your muscles and joints flexible in order to reach the state of physical comfort that comes from deep within your body. If your body is not comfortable, neither is your mind. Your mental state is directly connected to your physical well-being. Messages are constantly being sent from your body to the brain and back again.

You can become so accustomed to how it feels to be tense that only when you become aware of the difference between tension and relaxation can you do something about it. Shrug your shoulders, then just

Mind Relaxation

let them drop. This seems easy. But notice how often you are unaware and keep your shoulders shrugged during the day—talking on the phone, carrying a heavy bag, or sitting at the computer. Muscles and joints can become stiff simply from disuse. With a sedentary job or urban lifestyle— without a nearby mountain to climb—you often lose sight of your physical well-being. The yoga and stretching exercises shown in this book won't be the only flexibility regimen you'll need, but adding them to your bath will increase your comfort and range of movement.

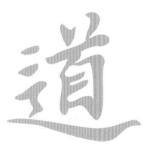

You can change the direction of your mind in half a second. When you realize that you are causing your own high stress level, try to quiet your thoughts. One way to do this is to imagine a huge STOP sign in front of you, and stop the chatter. Out of all the thoughts that go in and out of your mind, narrow the focus to only a few, then become aware of only one.

Meditations

Meditation can be done on many levels and can take many shapes and forms. It involves calling upon sights, feelings, sounds, and sensations that give you a sense of pleasure and comfort. When you guide yourself into calmness, your mind becomes more clear. Yoga is an inner practice. The first step is visualization. Because our sight is such a dominant sense, we are always visualizing something. In meditation, we choose a visual focus that will create a desired feeling.

Aromatherapy

Aromatherapy has been used for many years for its restorative effect on the body, mind, and spirit. In the practice of aromatherapy, different scents are used to bring about different moods. Smell, one of the strongest senses, can reawaken many pleasant memories and increase relaxation. Our olfactory receptors are closer to the brain than any of our other sensory organs. Engaging your sense of smell, along with your sight and sense of touch, will help your body respond to positive therapies more quickly.

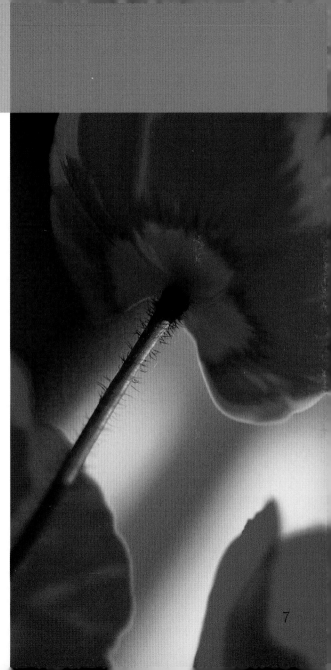

Yoga Breathing Practices

Breath is the life force; it is the bridge between your mind and your body. As natural as breathing is, we can do it more efficiently with practice. If you learn to slow down and regulate your breath, it will help you relax. Tension causes you to breathe at a faster and less even rate.

Lie comfortably in the tub and practice quiet breathing for a few moments. To begin, breathe in the manner that feels most natural. Breathe in through your nose to filter the air. Breathe out through your mouth to expel the air in a forceful exhalation. Make sure your throat, jaw, and facial muscles are relaxed. Also check that every part of your body is relaxed. Close your eyes and focus on the breath moving in and out. Breathe slowly and stay in a steady rhythm. Listen to the sound your breathing makes.

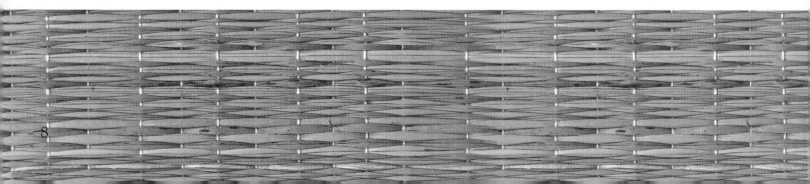

The Breathing Practices

Alternate Nostril Breathing

1. Begin with your index finger* blocking the right nostril; inhale through the left nostril.

2. Hold the inhalation for 4 counts, then use your thumb to block the left nostril; hold both nostrils closed for 4 counts.

*Each finger has a different energy. See page 22 for explanation.

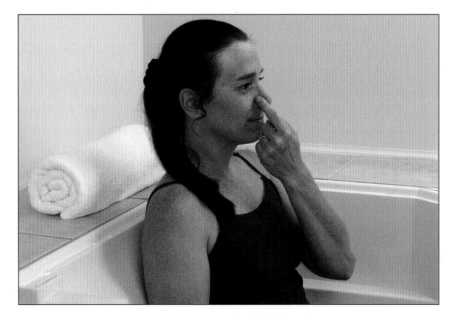

The Bathtub Yoga and Relaxation Book

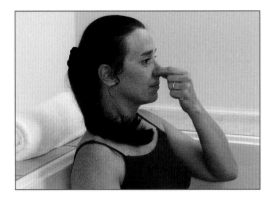

3. Release your index finger to open the right nostril, and exhale through it.

4. Now repeat the first 3 steps, beginning with the left nostril blocked and taking a deep breath through the right nostril.

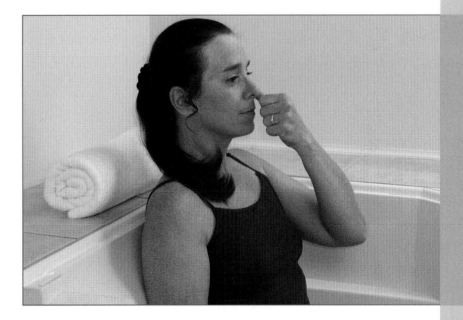

Supportive Breathing

1. Start by focusing on your breath. Be aware of how your lungs inflate, your body rises, and your abdominal muscles relax as you inhale.

2. Feel the sinking, heavy feeling and the contraction of the abdominal muscles as you exhale.

3. After a few rounds of breath, focus your attention on the sensation of sinking into the tub water. Feel the

parts of the body that touch the bottom of the tub, and with each exhalation feel those parts melting down into the tub floor.

4. When you feel completely relaxed, wiggle your toes and fingers, and start to slowly increase the rate of breathing.

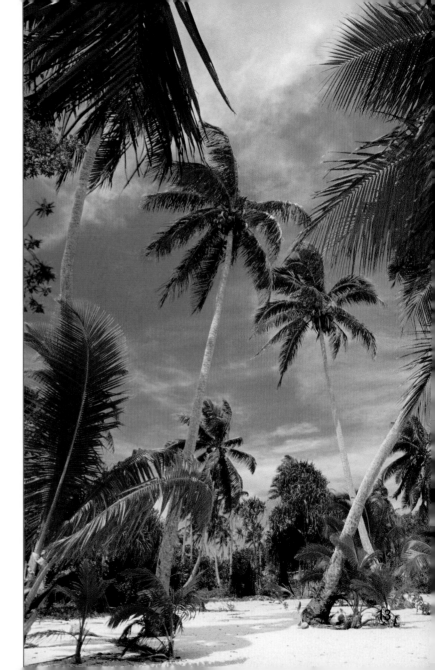

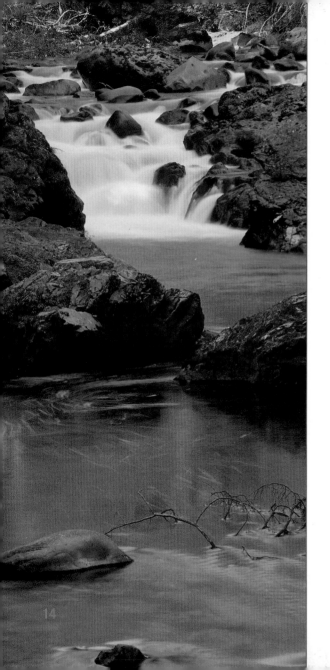

Four-Stage Abdominal Breathing

1. Keeping the abdominal muscles relaxed, inhale through your nose and fill your belly with air.

2. Continue the inhalation as you open your chest and fill your lungs with air.

3. Keep your lungs full with the rib cage lifted as you exhale first from your belly. Then pull in the abdominals to increase the force of the exhalation.

4. Complete the exercise by expelling all of the air in your lungs.

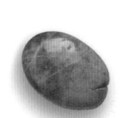

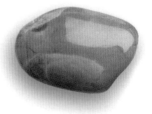

The Bathtub Yoga and Relaxation Book

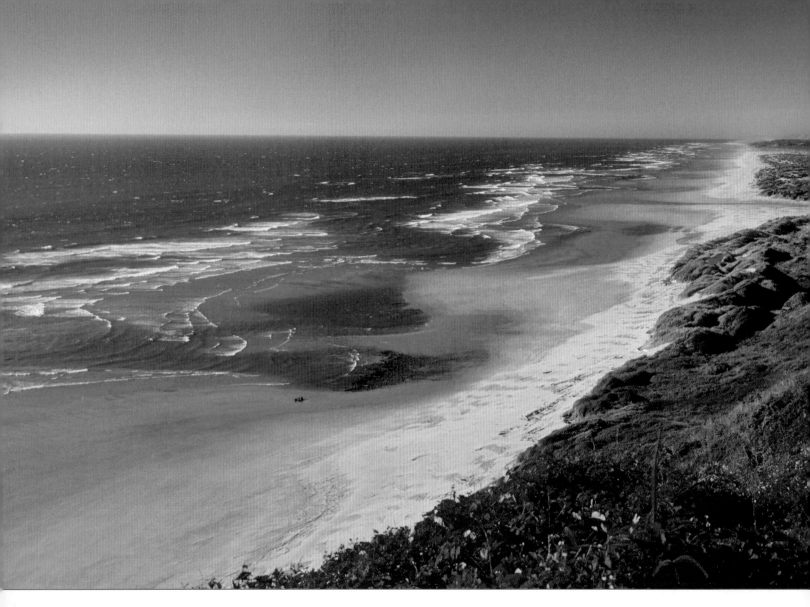

The Bathtub Yoga and Relaxation Book

Diaphragmatic Breathing

1. Inhale, relaxing the abdominal muscles. Feel your diaphragm push out and your ribs expand.

2. Exhale, contracting the abdominal muscles. The ribs close and the shoulders stay relaxed. Watch your belly rise and fall effort-lessly. Feel yourself riding the wave of your breath.

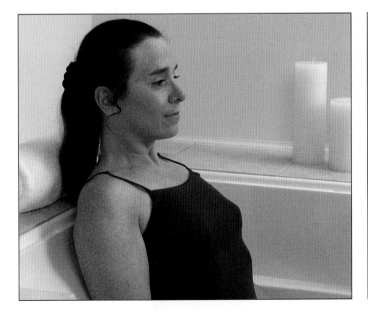
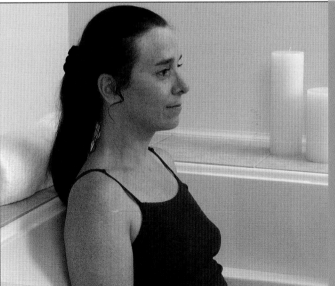

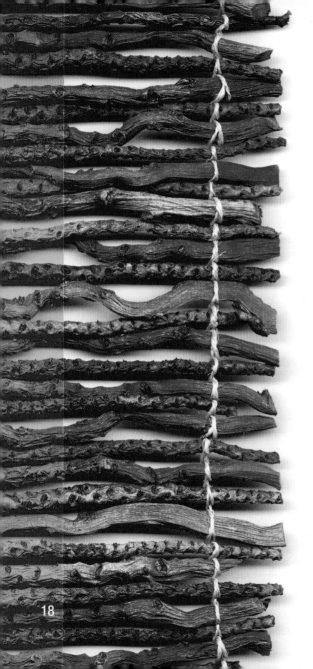

Step-by-Step Exhalation

1. Practice counting as you inhale and exhale slowly and deeply.

2. Begin with a count of 4 for the inhalation; hold 3 counts; then 4 counts for the exhalation. Let the breath out in steps; pause between each step.

3. With practice, lengthen the breath by increasing the counts and number of steps.

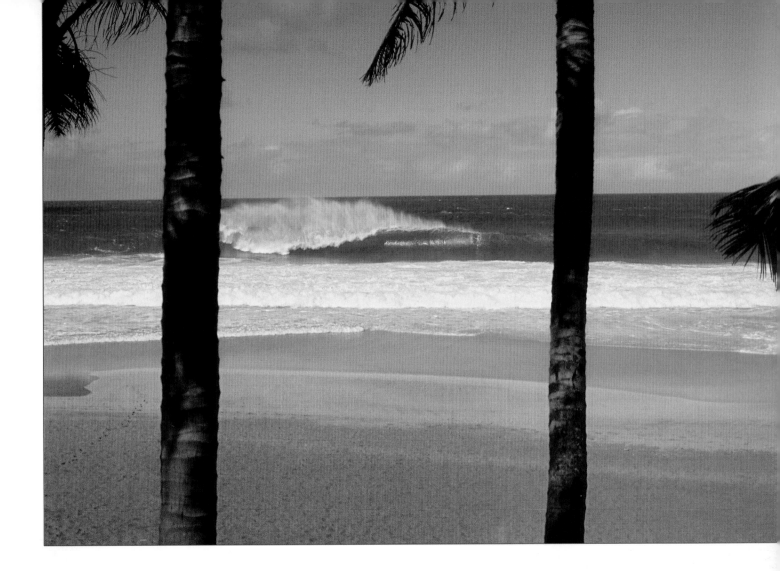

Body Relaxation

Water Yoga and Stretches

Yoga means union—uniting breath and movement to soothe and electrify the body and the mind. Traditional yoga postures are respectfully recreated here for the bathtub. Combined with the mental images of sea creatures, these exercises will free and refresh the spirit. Gentle yoga postures can be performed by everyone to relax the body. Clearing the mind with deep relaxation and meditation reduces stress and creates serenity and mental focus.

You can try using a rolled-up towel under your neck for additional comfort when you lie back to exercise. If you use one, wrap it in plastic to keep it dry.

Of course, as with any time you move around in a bathtub, *you must be sure not to slip.* Some tubs already have nonslip mats, but if not, we recommend you use one. They are easy to find and inexpensive to buy.

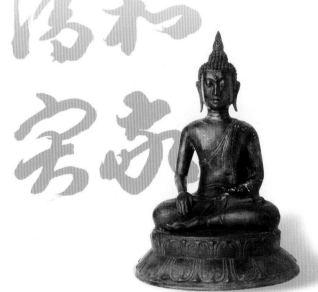

Water Yoga

This section is designed to balance and energize your body. You'll move in a comfortable way that promotes a fluid feeling from head to toe. Doing yoga in the water is peaceful and nurturing. These exercises are not demanding or challenging. The yoga-like moves and breathing practices will help transport you into a deeper state of relaxation. The deeper the rest, the greater the restoration of energy.

Chanting various syllables or words creates sound vibrations. A tiled bathroom has an energy of its own and is an interesting environment in which to magnify these vibrations. According to yoga teaching, sound vibrations open up the body's energy channels. When chanting the simple syllable "Om" or other sounds, you can feel vibrations through the whole thoracic cavity. Sounds that help you achieve a feeling of well-being are called mantras. They help to focus your mind, open the energy centers, and promote Shanti, the word for peace in Sanskrit (the ancient Indian language used in yoga teaching).

Yoga Positions, Chakras, and Other Energy Sources

According to ancient yoga practice, there are seven dynamic energy centers in the body called Chakras. The root of the word Chakra means wheel, and like wheels, they are always spinning. These seven centers draw energy from nature and the universe and adapt that energy for use within the body. Each Chakra affects different parts of the mind, body, and spirit. These bathtub practices will recharge and enhance the vitality of each Chakra.

The yoga postures and body positions in this section correspond to these centers. For example, The Whale (7th Chakra) corresponds to the Crown Chakra at the top of the head, similar to the blowhole on the top of a whale. We'll do a breathing exercise that blows away tension through the Crown Chakra.

Yoga practice encourages visualization and often animals are used to help the process, for example the cat, dog, and lion poses. We've chosen the sea creature that best correlates with each of the Chakras for you to use for your bathtub yoga practice.

Clam	Coccyx	1st
Mermaid	Sacral Plexus	2nd
Jellyfish	Solar Plexus	3rd
Otter	Heart Plexus	4th
Seal	Throat	5th
Squid	Third Eye	6th
Whale	Crown	7th

Following the 7 yoga sea creature positions is the Starfish Position, which uses traditional hand gestures called Mudras to complete the harmony of mind and body.

Neutral, Positive, and Negative Finger and Toe Energy

In an energy system, the goal is to balance opposing relationships. For example: The sun and moon work together in the same system. The sun gives outgoing "positive" yang energy. The moon has receptive "negative" yin energy and lights up because it receives the incoming energy from the sun.

Each finger and toe has a different energy:

Thumb and big toe	Neutral
Index finger and 2nd toe	Negative
Middle finger and 3rd toe	Positive
Ring finger and 4th toe	Negative
Little finger and 5th toe	Positive

Polarity System

According to the energy-based Polarity system, the 5 elements are the basic building blocks of all life. Each elemental energy is linked to a specific emotion and quality of being.

The fingers and toes correlate with these 5 elements:

Thumb and big toe	Ether	Nothingness—a creative neutral space
Index finger and 2nd toe	Air	Thinking—ideas
Middle finger and 3rd toe	Fire	Purposefulness
Ring finger and 4th toe	Water	Sensuality
Little finger and 5th toe	Earth	Stability

7 salutory effects of bathing:

- *relaxation of body*
- *avoidance of cold*
- *avoidance of pain*
- *avoidance of chills*
- *avoidance of fever*
- *avoidance of filth*

and refreshing the body and clearing the mind

JAPANESE SUTRA ON BATHS AND BATHING FOR THE CLERGY

The Bathtub Yoga and Relaxation Book

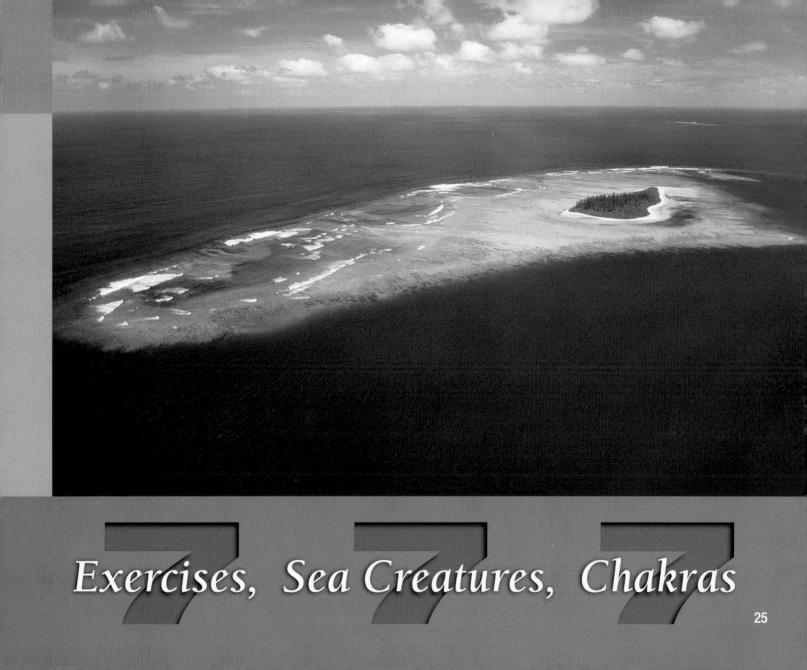

Exercises, Sea Creatures, Chakras

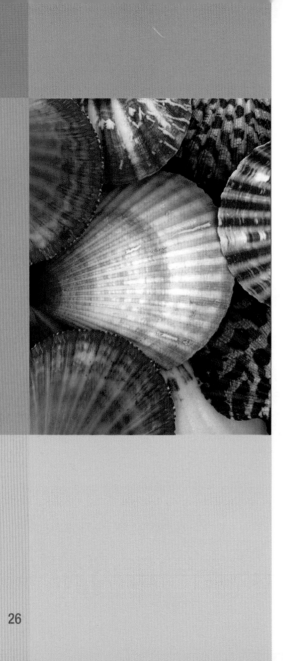

The Clam

1st Chakra—Coccyx

Curve your body into the shape of a clam shell, and wiggle at the hinge.

1. Curl forward and bring your right knee toward your chest.

2. Place your left hand on top of your bent right knee and your right hand around your right buttock.

3. Breathe fully and deeply as you shift your coccyx (tailbone) from side to side. Keep the left leg straight out and against the tub front for support. Alternate sides.

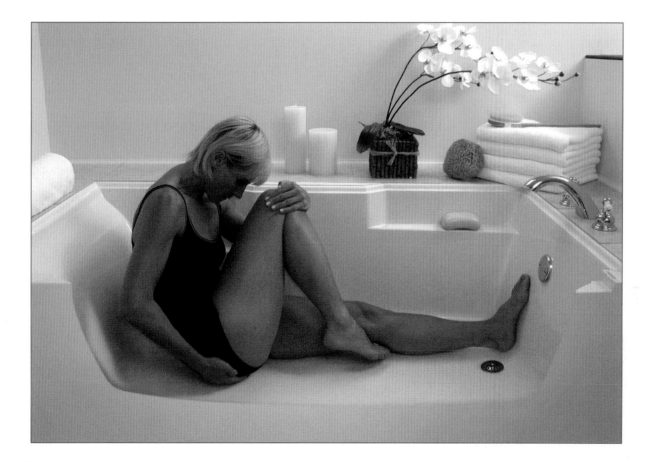

Body Relaxation—Water Yoga

The Mermaid

2nd Chakra—Sacral Plexus

Sitting upon a rock, be on the lookout for all sailors and ships.

1. Sit with both legs straight out and balance your weight on both sit bones.

2. Bend your right knee, placing your foot solidly on the tub floor on the outside of your left leg. Curl your left hand around the bent knee, and keep your right hand on the tub floor for support.

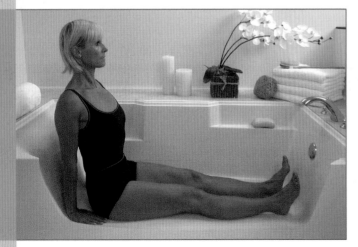
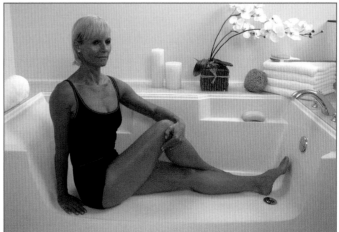

The Bathtub Yoga and Relaxation Book

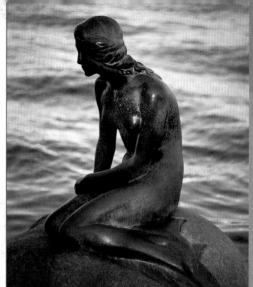

3. Inhale as you rotate your upper body and look over your right shoulder. Exhale and let your body sink into the water and relax.

4. Repeat on the other side.

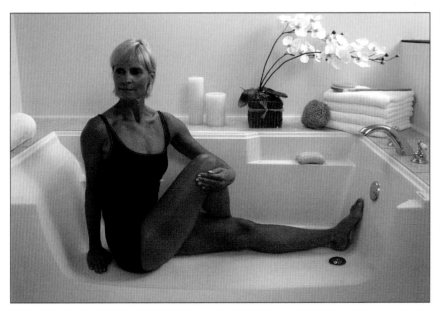

Body Relaxation—Water Yoga

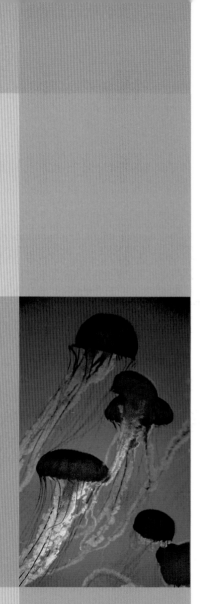

The Jellyfish

3rd Chakra—Solar Plexus

Float on top of a wave just like the inflated jellyfish does.

1. Sit up and put both hands behind your hips, fingers pointed in.

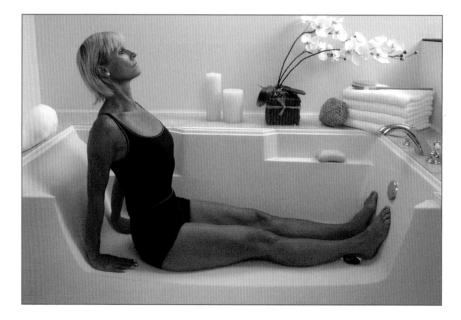

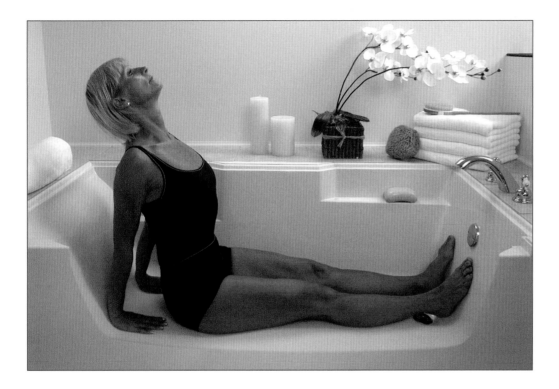

2. Anchor your feet against the front of the tub. Breathe deeply and lift your chest.

3. Inhale and expand your chest; then exhale and use the strength in your arms to hold the position for 15 seconds.

Body Relaxation—Water Yoga

The Otter

4th Chakra—Heart Plexus

Feel like an otter floating on its back, paws together and enjoying an abalone shell.

1. Lie back and start with your legs straight. Slowly bend the right knee out to the side, and bring the sole of that foot to rest against the inner knee (or calf or thigh) of your left leg.

2. Inhale deeply and bring your hands together near your heart, palm against palm into a prayer pose. Exhale and open the door of your

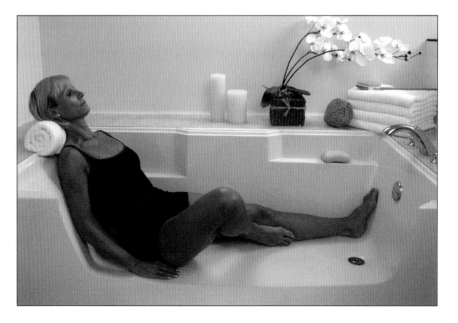

The Bathtub Yoga and Relaxation Book

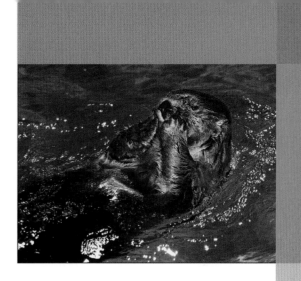

heart as you visualize a bright, shining star that radiates pure white light throughout your body.

3. Slowly straighten the right leg, and return your arms to your sides. Repeat with the other leg.

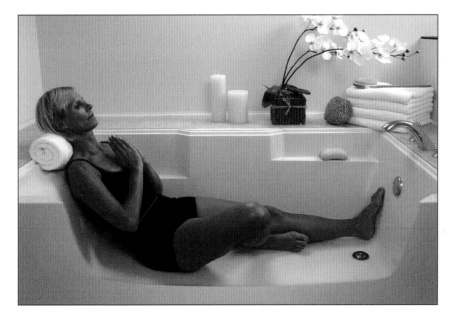

The Seal

5th Chakra—Throat

The undulating seal emits a throaty sound while calling to its mate.

1. "Ocean Breathing": Lie back and tilt your head back a bit to open up the throat. Practice saying the sound "Ha" out loud with your mouth open.

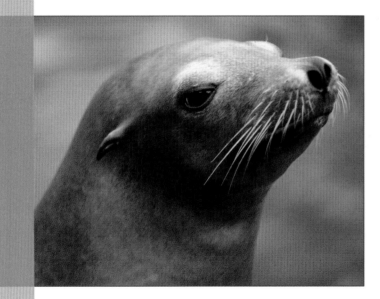

2. Now keep your mouth closed and voice quiet. Inhale and think a Ha sound; exhale with a silent Ha sound, dragging your breath deep into your throat.

3. The vibration in your throat opens the power of the voice and creates a sound like the waves of a peaceful ocean.

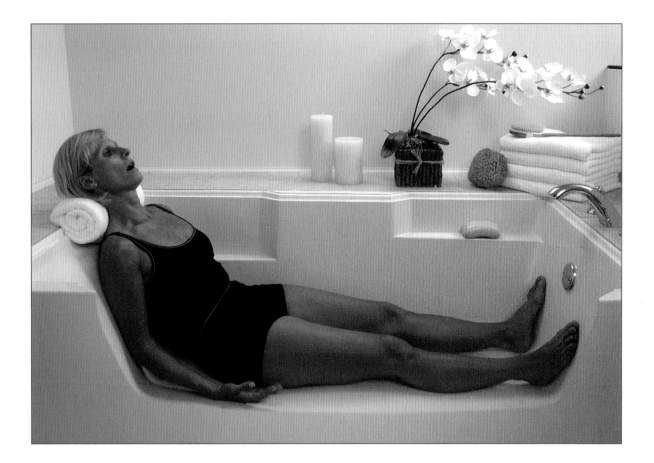

The Squid

6th Chakra—Third Eye

Focus on the squid's sharp eye, remarkably similar to that of humans.

1. Lie back. Keep your mouth closed and practice a humming sound.

2. Inhale through both nostrils and visualize the third eye on your forehead, directly between your eyebrows. With your mouth closed, exhale slowly, making a humming sound, and feel your eyebrows grow long.

3. Keep humming until there's no breath left and you feel the third eye space between your eyebrows broaden and relax.

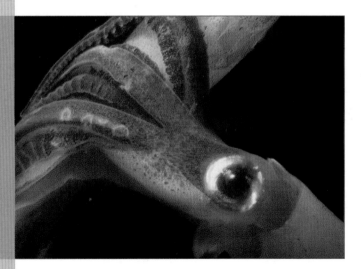

The Bathtub Yoga and Relaxation Book

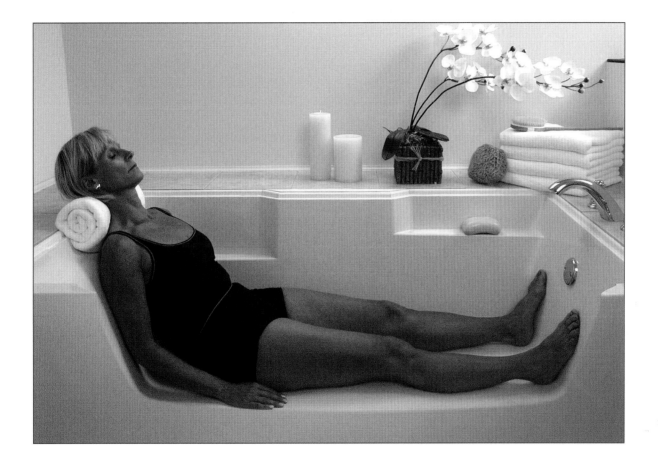

Body Relaxation—Water Yoga

The Whale

7th Chakra—Crown

Breathe away tension as if through the blowhole on the top of a whale.

1. Lie on your belly. Bend your arms with your hands on the tub floor, and point your fingers forward. Bend your knees and rest your feet on the rim of the tub.

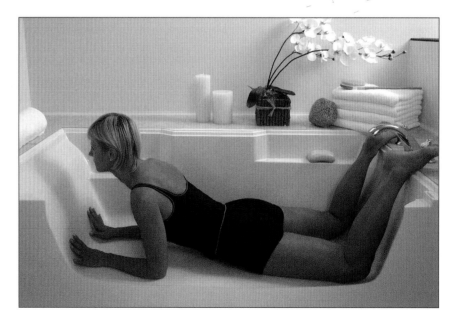

The Bathtub Yoga and Relaxation Book

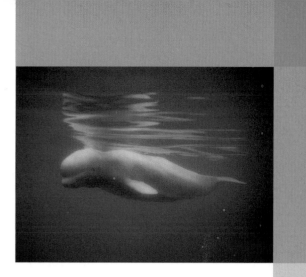

2. Inhale and stretch upward with the crown of your head; exhale through the imaginary blowhole at the top of the crown, and blow out your stress. Visualize a shower of white light coming right through that spot.

3. Relax and lower your body.

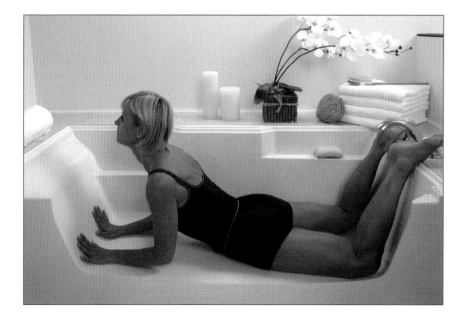

Starfish Position

To help you relax and achieve a feeling of calmness, borrow from the ancient, spiritual method of focusing on the Hara. The Hara is at the center of your belly, about an inch lower than your naval. Start your breath at that point and concentrate on how relaxing it feels. Add traditional yoga finger and hand gestures called Mudras to help you focus. The fingers possess both positive outgoing yang energy and receptor incoming yin energy. When these energies are balanced, your vitality is restored. The finger and hand pressure connects with different areas in the body and brain.

Just as a starfish lies flat and burrows down upon the sand, lie comfortably in the tub with your arms to the side. Breathe slowly and deeply, in through your nose and out through pursed lips. Pause in between each breath. With each breath, imagine a new beginning, a new possibility.

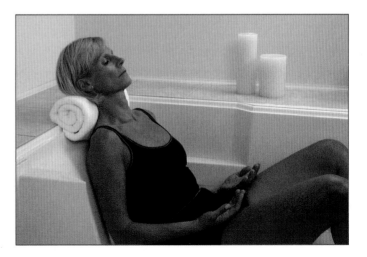

The Bathtub Yoga and Relaxation Book

1. Hold your palms open and facing up to receive energy from the universe.

2. Hold your palms open and facing up with thumbs touching your index finger to complete the energy circle.

3. Rest your hands at the Hara, palms facing up. Rest your left hand on your right palm. Let your thumbs touch to circulate the yin and yang energies. Yin and yang are opposing but complementary energies in the universe. The female yin is passive and represents the heavens, the moon, the night, and the autumn. Its symbol, the tiger, is unfathomable. The male yang is active and grounded and represents the sun, the day, and the spring. Its symbol, the dragon, is assertive. We achieve our sense of balance when these forces work together.

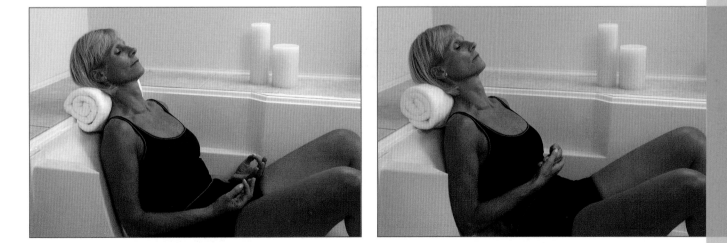

Water Stretches

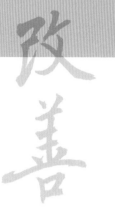

Stretching is a must to maintain supple joints. You probably already use a bath or shower to alleviate stiffness. The warm water relaxes your muscles and makes you feel better.

Stretching in the bath is an easy way to increase circulation and warm up the muscles. Cold muscles do not stretch as effectively as warmed up ones.

Stretching helps your muscles resist stress by keeping them elongated and relaxed. When you balance tension with relaxation, muscles remain strong, flexible and pain free.

Putting a rolled towel underneath your neck keeps the trapezius muscle—the one across your upper back and neck—relaxed and stretched. This is the exact spot where tension often gets trapped. Is it coincidental that "trap" is the first syllable of trapezius?

The Stretches

Neck Lengthener

Shoulder Circles

Hamstring Stretch

Thigh Stretch

Spine Flexibility

Hip Release

Wrist Flexibility

Finger Stretch

Ankle Mobility

Toe Mobility

Be aware of how your body feels as it's moving. Learn to feel which muscles are working as a way to increase mental focusing.

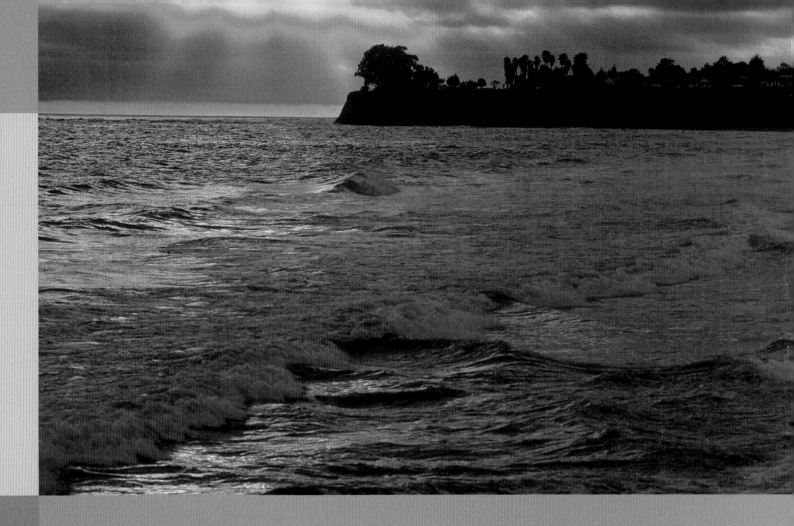

The Stretches

The Neck Lengthener

1. Sit back with both legs straight out.

2. With your left hand at the back of your head and your right hand on your right shoulder, turn your head slowly and look over your right shoulder. Keep your shoulders pulled down. Feel how the warm water makes it easier to keep your shoulders down.

3. Turn your head back to center and repeat to the other side. Pause and repeat 3 times.

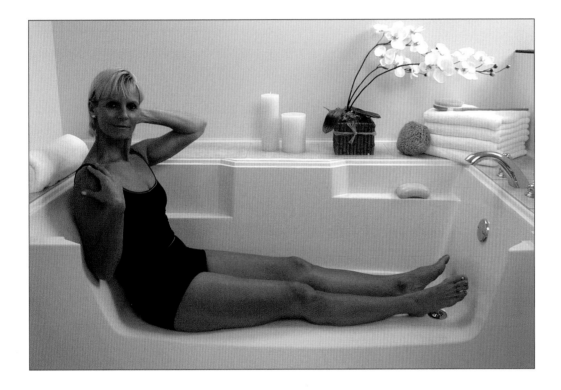

Body Relaxation—Water Stretches

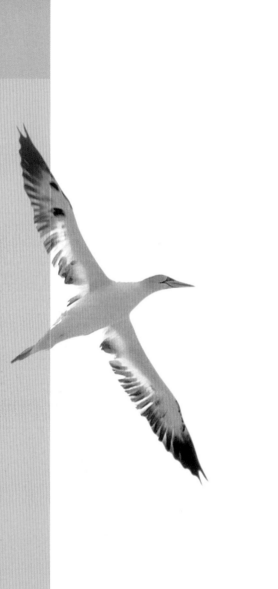

Shoulder Circles

1. Sit with your legs bent comfortably and your body weight tilting forward of your tailbone. Keep your body connected to the tub floor.

2. Bend your arms and place your fingertips on your shoulders.

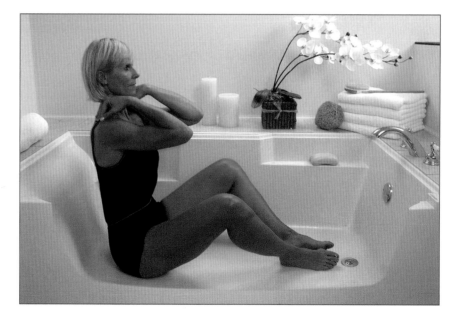

The Bathtub Yoga and Relaxation Book

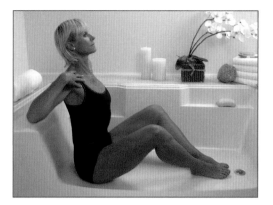

3. Slowly make backward circles. Feel the chest muscles stretching and the shoulder blades move in towards the spine. Pause and repeat 3 times.

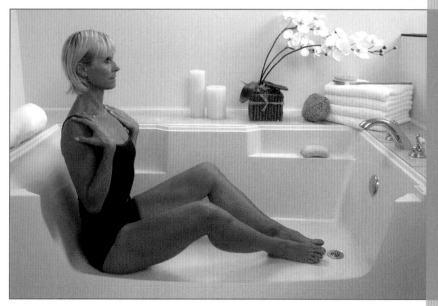

Hamstring Stretch

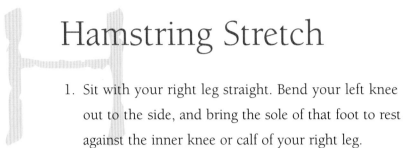

1. Sit with your right leg straight. Bend your left knee out to the side, and bring the sole of that foot to rest against the inner knee or calf of your right leg.

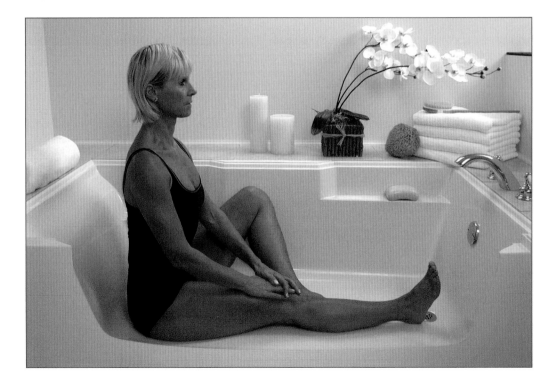

The Bathtub Yoga and Relaxation Book

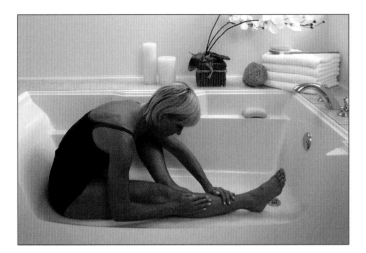 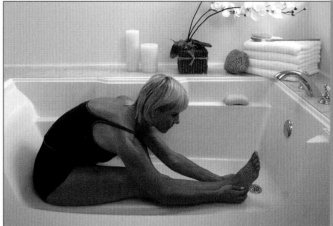

2. Slowly curve your head and shoulders down towards your right knee.

3. Slide your hands along your right leg toward your foot in a slow count of 5, and feel the hamstring stretch along the back of the thigh. Use your breath and the warmth of the water to increase the stretch.

4. Roll up, change legs, and repeat on the other side.

Thigh Stretch

1. Sit up and bend your right knee with your foot on the tub floor.

2. Lean back with your left hand on the tub floor as you turn your right thigh inward.

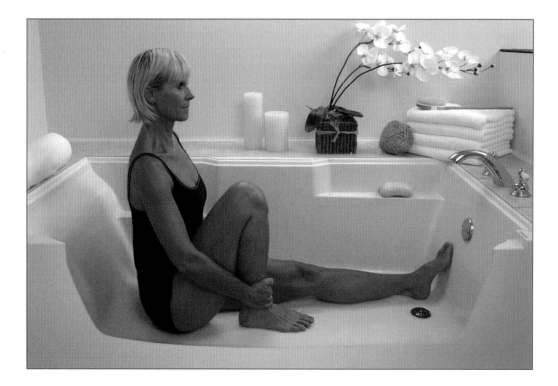

The Bathtub Yoga and Relaxation Book

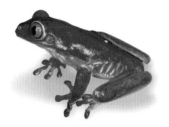

3. Hold your right ankle and feel the stretch along the top of your thigh.

4. Change legs.

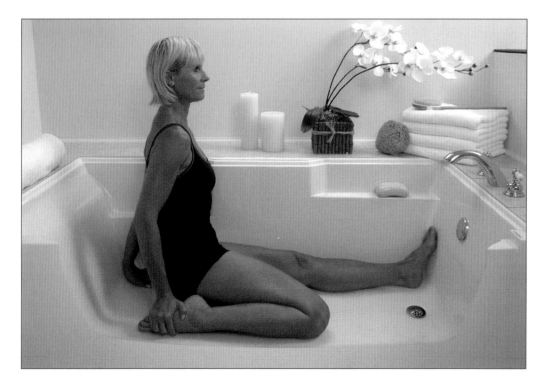

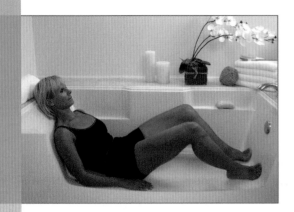

Spine Flexibility

1. Lean back with your legs straight out. Raise up and rest on your elbows. Bend your knees, keeping your feet securely on the tub floor.

2. Lift your hips very slightly off the tub floor.

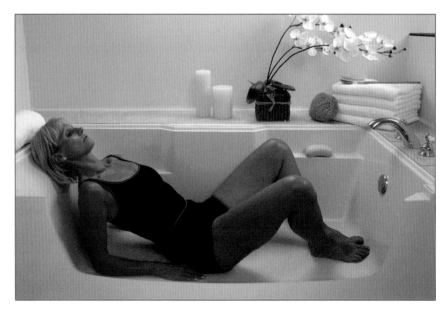

The Bathtub Yoga and Relaxation Book

3. Slowly curl and uncurl your back in a wave-like motion to stretch your spine.

4. Slowly lower your hips back down to the tub floor.

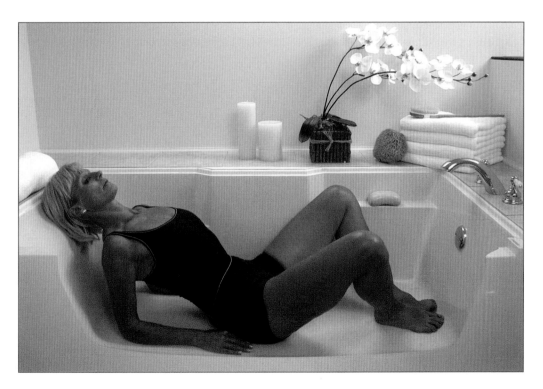

Hip Release

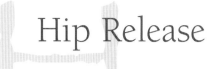

1. Sit back with your legs straight out.

2. Inhale and bring your left knee towards your chest. Keep your right foot against the front of the tub to hold your balance.

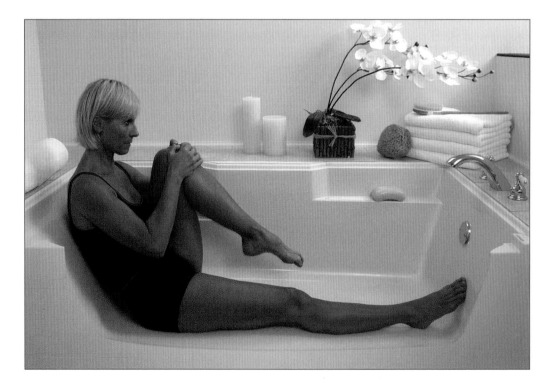

The Bathtub Yoga and Relaxation Book

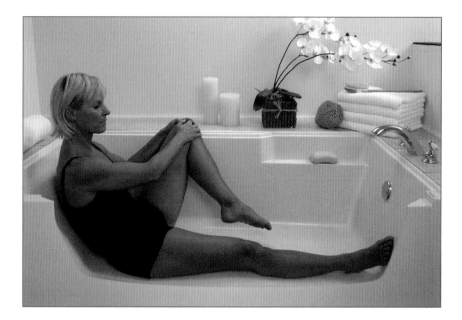

3. Hold the top of your left knee and slowly trace 3 circles in each direction. Feel the full range of motion in the hip joint, the place where the thigh bone meets the pelvis.

4. Change legs. Pause and repeat 3 times.

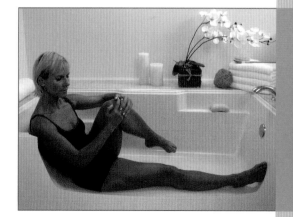

Wrist Flexibility

The starting position for each of the four wrist exercises is the same. Do 5 slow repetitions of each exercise.

Starting position: Either lie back or sit with your legs bent comfortably and your body weight tilting forward of your tailbone. Bend your arms at a right angle and keep your elbows close to your waist.

1. Use imaginary resistance as you slowly bend your wrist down and hold for 5 seconds. Return and repeat.

2. Flex your wrists up and hold for 5 seconds. Return and repeat.

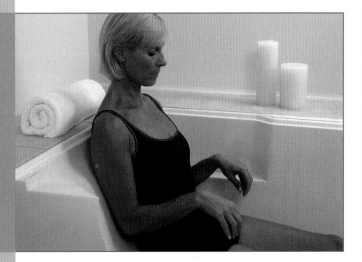 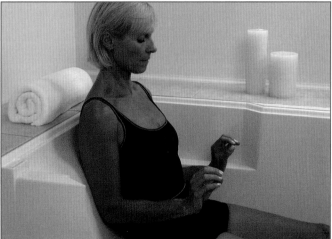

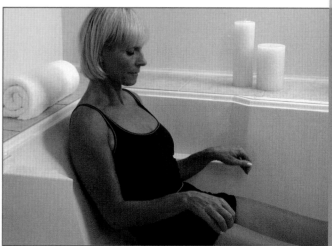

3. Keep your wrists on the same plane and slowly move them from side to side like windshield wipers. *(continued)*

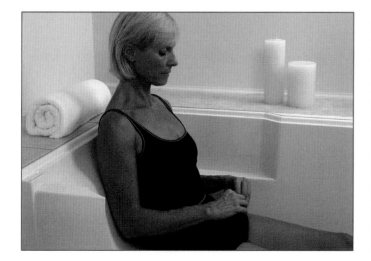

Body Relaxation—Water Stretches

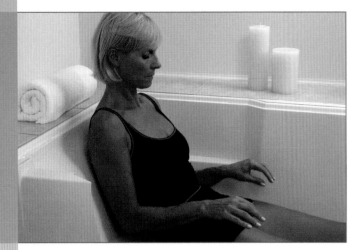
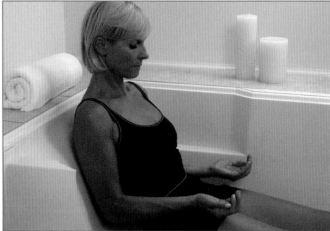

4. Begin with your wrists and forearms
   facing down, and slowly turn them so
   they face up. Turn back and repeat.

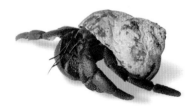

The Bathtub Yoga and Relaxation Book

Finger Stretch

1. Lie back with both legs stretched straight out.

2. Stretch both arms forward. Grasp the fingertips of your right hand with your left hand.

3. Gently pull your fingers closer to your body; then press your fingers and hand down.

4. Repeat with the other hand.

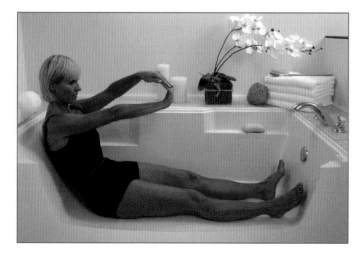
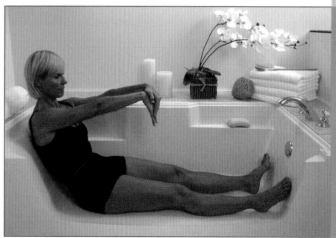

Ankle Mobility

The starting position for each of the 3 ankle exercises is the same. Do 5 slow repetitions of each exercise.

Starting Position: Sit with your legs straight out.

1. Stretch your heels out, flex your feet, and bring the toes straight up. In five counts, press down one section of the foot at a time:

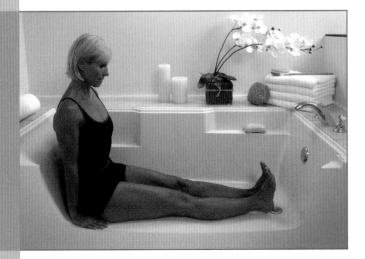
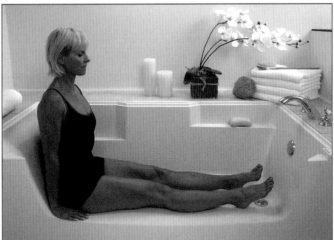

The Bathtub Yoga and Relaxation Book

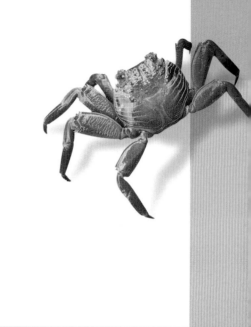

- press the heel forward (toes spread and up)

- press down on the arch (toes up)

- press down on the ball of the foot (toes up)

- press down on the top of the foot

- point the toes down

- curl the toes and slowly return to starting position to repeat. *(continued)*

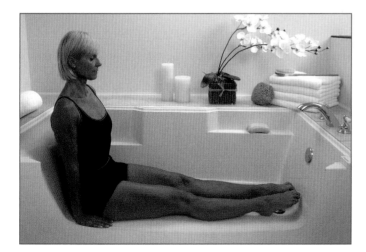

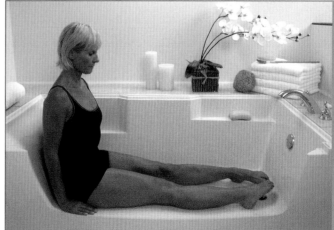

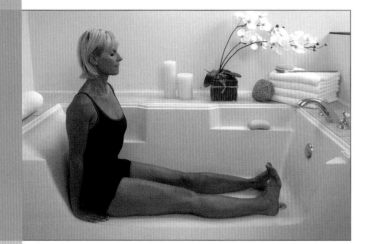 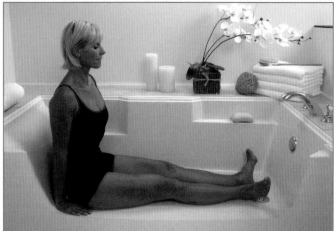

2. Press your feet down and point your toes.

• Keep your heels in place as you bring your big toes together to form an upside-down "V."

• Feel the arches pulling up, and hold for five seconds. Relax and repeat.

The Bathtub Yoga and Relaxation Book

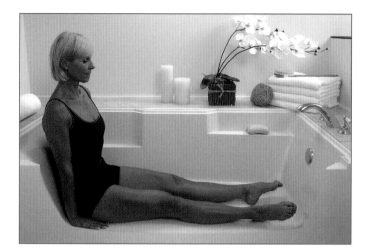
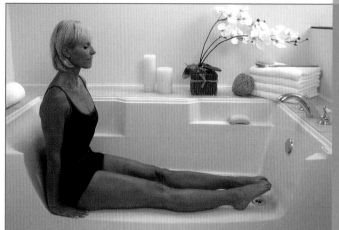

3. Foot circles. Turn in the toes, press the ankles
   down, and trace circles with the feet.

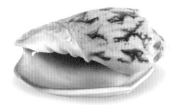

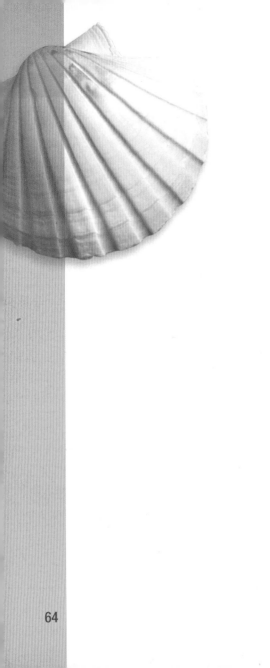

Toe mobility

1. Lie back with both legs straight out. Work one foot at a time.

2. Imagine a golf ball placed underneath your toes. Curl your toes over the ball and hold for a slow

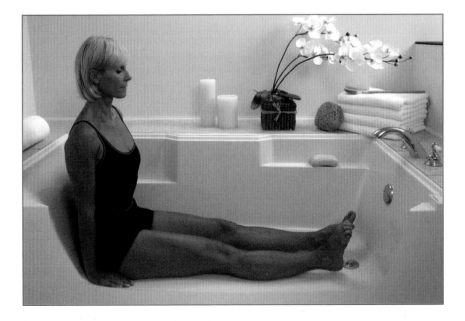

The Bathtub Yoga and Relaxation Book

count of 5. Release and repeat 5 times; change feet.

3. Imagine no more ball. Press the balls of the feet forward and spread the toes wide apart. Repeat 5 times.

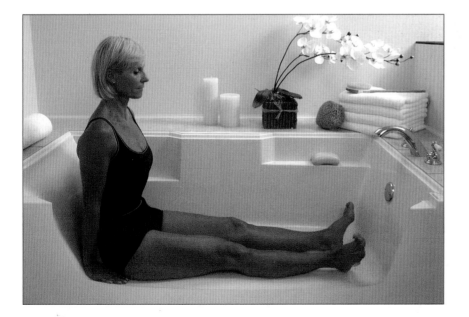

Mind Relaxation

Meditation

There is no right way to meditate, only the way that feels good to you.

The aim of meditation is to create a focused awareness in which the "chatter" within your mind gives way to stillness and inner peace. Place yourself in the stillness of meditation.

You know if your mind is working overtime and you need to reduce your stress level. You can tell if your body feels tense and needs to relax. A warm bath is the perfect place to unwind your mind and body.

You should experiment to find the positions that are most comfortable for you to do your meditations. A rolled-up towel, covered with plastic, is effective when placed beneath the neck for support. Depending on the shape of your tub, you may want to place your hands on either side of your neck to hold the towel in place and to give your neck more support. This also allows you to sink into whatever position feels best.

If your legs begin to feel uncomfortable, here's an easy way to rest and stretch them. Bend the left leg at the knee and cross it over the right leg. Rest your left arm on the side of the tub. Cross your right arm over your left leg, and rest the wrist on your left knee. When you have eased any tension or discomfort in the left leg, change position and repeat on the other side.

The first step in stress reduction is to use your mind to develop concentration and focus. Here's a way to eliminate distractions and let go of all the things you're thinking about.

Meditation

Sample Focused Relaxation Exercise

Focused relaxation feels wonderful in the tub. Use your breath to structure your relaxation. Focus on one group of muscles at a time, and think of sending the breath to that spot. With each exhalation, breathe away the tension. Sense the "letting go" of your body. Close your eyes and block out all external stimuli.

Begin with the toes and end with the head, in the following order:

- Right foot
- Left foot
- Right leg
- Left leg
- Hips and abdomen
- Buttocks
- Shoulder blades and shoulders
- Right arm
- Left arm
- Neck and head
- Muscles around the eyes and mouth

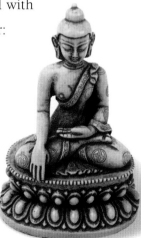

Create each day anew by clothing yourself with wisdom and love,
and placing yourself in the heart of Mother Nature.

MORIKEI UESHIBA,
FOUNDER OF AKIDO
O-SENSEI'S COLLECTED TALES "THE ART OF PEACE"

Mental focusing teaches you how to identify with the spaces between your thoughts rather than only the thoughts themselves. As you meditate, be aware of how the breathing helps. The pause at the end of each exhalation is the "space". . . the "letting go" of tension.

We suggest the use of affirmations to enhance the meditating experience. Affirmations come from words you create to feel better. Use motivational words that inspire you. They can be powerful statements about any part of your life.

We've created the following meditations, some with affirmations. As you become familiar with using them, feel free to create your own statements. You can use affirmations as a way to honor your spirituality, handle challenges, build confidence, make choices, help form a positive belief system, or for many other situations. There are limitless ways to establish a richer life.

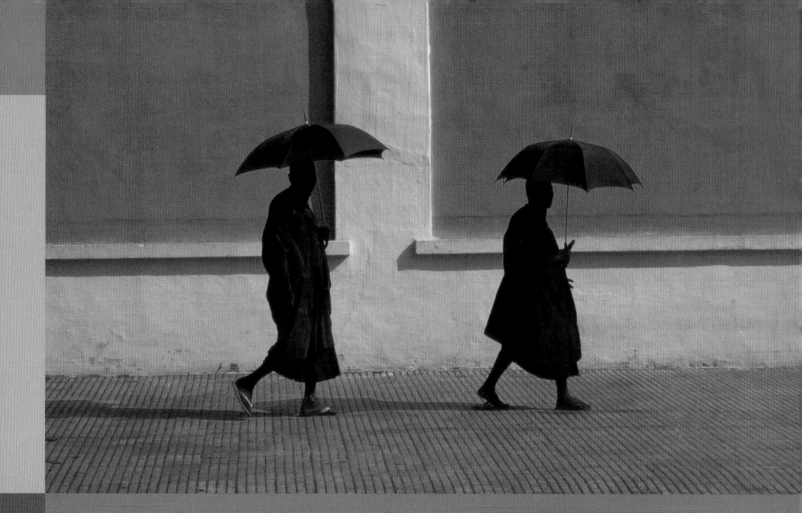

The Meditations

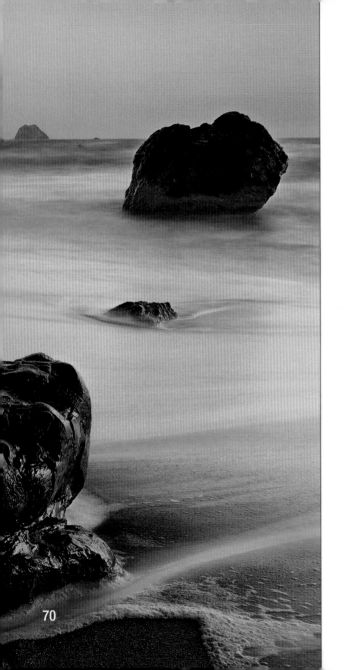

Gentle Meditation

1. Lie comfortably and take a deep breath. Scan your body to make sure that every part of you feels physically relaxed.

2. As you breathe, imagine that you're in the most beautiful place in nature.

3. Now imagine that the qualities of your landscape—the air, the waves of the ocean, or the petals of the flowers—are like a fine mist showering your whole body with every inhalation.

4. With each exhalation, this energy feeds into every cell of your being, loving, nurturing, and embracing you. Breathe in this energy as long as you can.

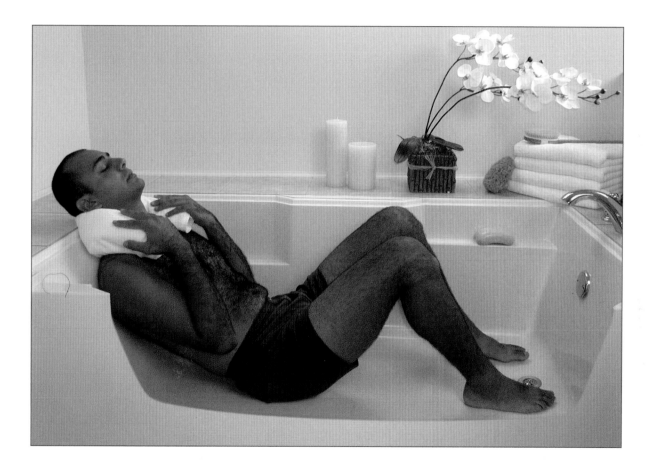

The Bathtub Yoga and Relaxation Book

Energizing Meditation

1. Lie back and take a deep breath. Be sure that every part of you feels relaxed.

2. Quietly say to yourself: "As I breathe in, I am energizing my body and my mind. As I breathe out, I smile into this moment, which is the only moment, feeling well cared for in the warm water. I feel protected by a divine bright light that is circling all around me now. I surrender, body and soul, to this ultimate experience of peace within."

Spirituality surrounds you, waiting for you to tap into it.

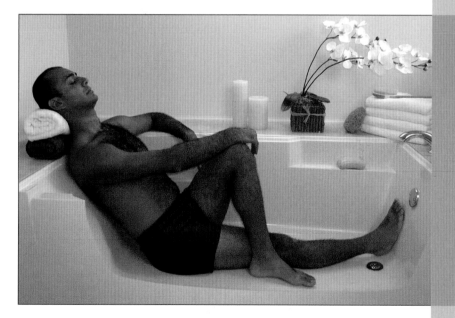

Mindfulness Meditation

1. Make yourself comfortable and observe how good it feels to be where you are here and now.

2. Silently say to yourself, "I am now still," and think it again, "I am now still."

3. Become aware of the length of your body, the space it occupies, and the presence of your heart far away from your feet.

4. Begin to enjoy the perfect symmetry of your body, from right to left shoulder; from right to left arm; from right to left hip; from right to left buttock; from right to left leg; from right to left foot. As you experience this deep sense of well-being, connect to your breath, the source of life. Begin to feel the air tickling your nostrils; feel the breath filling your whole body with energy, life force, and new life.

5. As you continue to go deeper and deeper into relaxation, think to yourself silently, " I am now calm and relaxed," and then say it again.

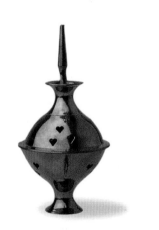

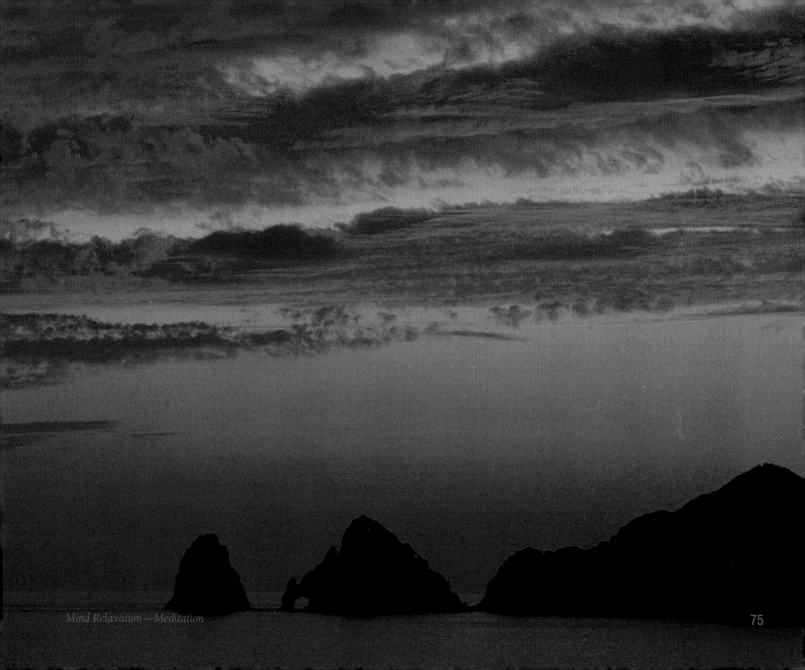

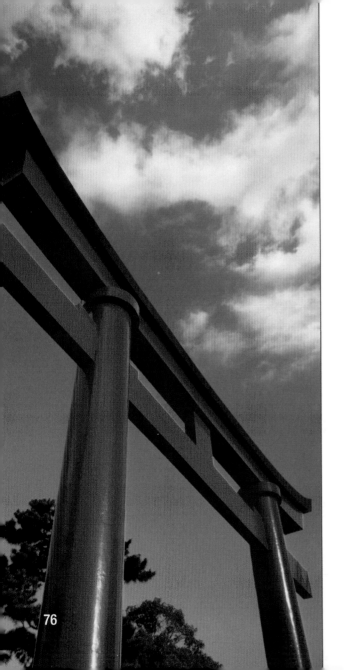

Wisdom Meditation

1. Either sitting or lying comfortably, think "I am still now," and think it again.

2. Feel perfect balance between your left side and your right side.

3. Imagine a magnificent lake—a perfectly still, tranquil lake without a ripple disturbing the surface—and try to sit without a single thought disturbing your mind.

4. As you observe this lake, say to yourself, "I am now focused and calm; calm and focused." Continue to focus on your breathing, feeling each breath effortlessly and peacefully entering your nostrils and filling your whole body up with new life force and strength.

5. As you continue to feel more calm and more relaxed, look around the lake. Notice the trees, the sky, and the presence of a quaint wooden cabin.

6. Take a walk towards the front porch and walk inside. Notice the presence of a stranger; it is a sage, a wise person of limitless knowledge and compassion. Know that this person is very concerned about your welfare and eager to help you. Just introduce yourself and ask a question about an issue that is on your mind. Allow yourself to be receptive. Be open to whatever answer comes to you.

7. After several minutes, express gratitude to this person and take leave. Walk out of the cabin, look at the lake for the last time, and return refreshed, peaceful, and wise.

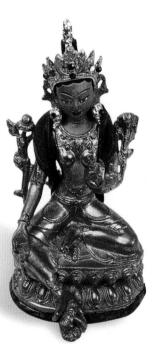

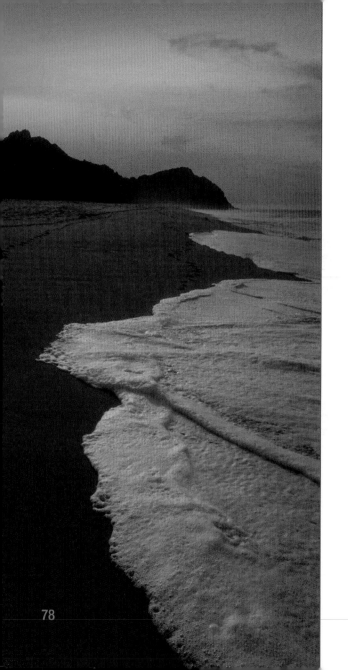

Healing Meditation

1. Lie back with your knees bent and feet flat on the tub floor. Imagine the earth beneath you and roots (like a tree) growing underneath your feet.

2. Now imagine your head floating up towards the sky as you attach it to an invisible string.

3. So here you are between earth and heaven. Perfect yin and yang balance. Appreciate this exquisite experience and smile. Smile at this perfect moment which is the only moment we have.

4. As you keep smiling, notice how your facial muscles begin to release tension from your forehead, eyes, cheeks, and chin.

5. Imagine yourself now surrounded by a circle of divine white light. As the circle of light surrounds you, it protects you against any negative energy.

The Bathtub Yoga and Relaxation Book

6. Complete this experience by imagining a shower of golden light coming down from the sky and cleansing your aura, making it vibrant. You now receive light from inside out and outside in. You are pure light and divine energy. You are healed.

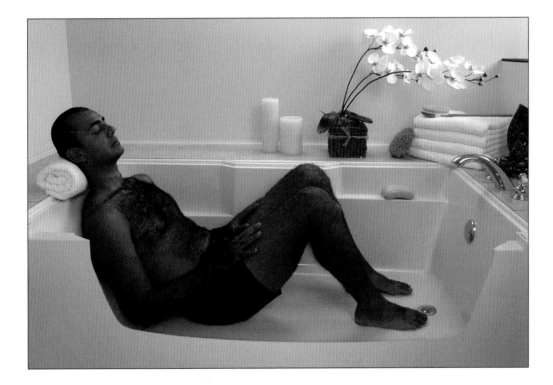

I have no faith in medicines.
My remedies are fasting
and the warm bath.

EMPEROR NAPOLEON BONAPARTE

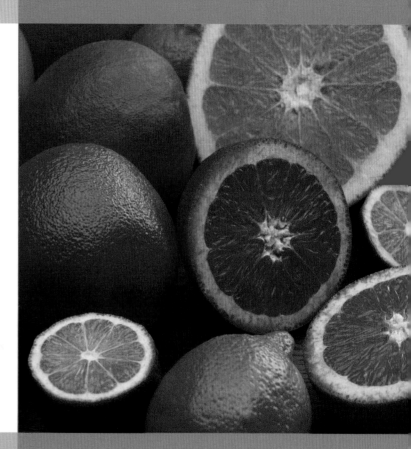

Aromatherapy

A warm bath is pleasing and relaxing by itself. However, you can add desirable scents into your bathing time with candles, natural ingredients, flower petals, or aromatic oils. Scents, sounds, and colors all evoke feelings. Choosing the right scent can put you in a better mood. We associate pleasure with whatever makes us feel good.

More and more people are using natural ingredients to promote a variety of benefits. Many of these products can be found right in your own home or at a nearby market. Some are energizing; others are calming. These are some of the products you can add to your bath water to release the scent; use about a handful or a cup.

Sliced lemons, limes, oranges	Energizing
Milk	Smoothing and nourishing
Shaved ginger	Cleansing
Vanilla extract	Comforting
Oatmeal	Toning and soothing

Oatmeal baths and facials can tighten the skin and also soothe irritation. One friend used this combination to soothe her itching, and she swears by it! Put dry oatmeal in a blender to crush flakes into a powdery form. Put this in the bath water. Make a paste from the oatmeal and water, and rub it very gently on your body.

Cucumbers	Cooling

You can lie comfortably back in the bath and cover each eye with a chilled slice of cucumber for a relaxing eye mask.

Baking soda	Softens skin
Epsom salts	Healing

Soaking in epsom salts, like a swim in the ocean, helps cuts and scratches heal, lowers blood pressure, and helps muscles release.

Some people believe that placing salt water in a room keeps negativity away. Just as the mind is impressed with what other people say and do, the aura or energy field around the body also receives impressions. These impressions need to be cleansed so that we stay centered. A combination of $1/2$ cup of baking soda and $1/2$ cup of epsom salts in the bath makes you feel refreshed and relaxed from the inside out. (This is especially helpful for those in service industries who are in close contact with other people all day.)

Add rose petals or petals from any other flower whose fragrance you like. For example, the scent of lavender petals is very relaxing. Take a handful and sprinkle the petals throughout the bath water.

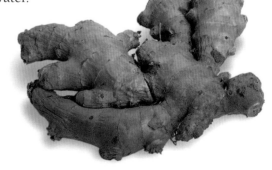

There's a wide array of aromatherapy combinations to choose from. Try out different scents and aromatic oils to see what you like. Aromatic essential oils are extracted from plants, herbs, and flowers. You can place a few drops of oil into your bath water. Have you noticed how nice various kitchen herbs smell? Sprinkle a handful of dried herbs in warm bath water, and you'll smell the essence of the herb. You can grow your own herb plants or buy herbs in your local nursery or health food store. Make a bundle and hang them upside down to dry. Then gently take the herbs off the stem and crumble them in your hands to release the smell of the herb.

Herbalists suggest using these aromatherapy oils in combination or alone for the following satisfying effects:

Rosewood and ylang-ylang	Nourishing
Patchouli and rosewood	Sexually stimulating
Rosemary and mint	Physically stimulating
Sweet lavender	Relaxing
Eucalyptus	Mentally stimulating and energizing
Juniper	Clearing/digestive
Peppermint	Circulation

The bath is a quiet, comforting, and natural place to relax and feel good. You'll be surprised how easy it is to create a daily ritual of getting into the tub, putting in a few drops of a pleasantly scented oil, and meditating. Taking care of your body contributes as much to your general well-being as anything.

Conclusion

We've come to the end of *The Bathtub Yoga and Relaxation Book,* but it's just the beginning of a new approach to wellness. Most people enjoy taking a warm, relaxing bath, and we hope we've showed you some new ways to enhance your bath experience. Remember, this is a special time for you.

Why? The relationship you have with yourself is one of the first—and the most important. Don't hesitate to love and honor yourself. Self-esteem fuels positive behavior which leads to greater satisfaction in life. This esteem is a learned belief, a learned attitude, and it means having confidence. Don't be afraid to compliment yourself. When you talk to yourself, say the same encouraging things you would say to a friend.

Many of you already include exercise in your life. Some of you may not. For all of you, the mild postures and stretching this book teaches you to do in the bath will heighten your body awareness. They will help you to feel more connected to your inner self and to the person you really are. Knowing how to use your body will also give you increased confidence.

We hope *The Bathtub Yoga and Relaxation Book* has inspired you to *take more time out for yourself.* Combining stretching with relaxation—the most valuable habit you can develop—will give you real and lasting benefits. The enjoyment you get when taking care of

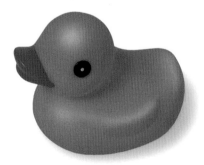

your body is the best motivation. Feel comfortable as you exercise. If an exercise doesn't feel right, you won't get the benefits you want and you may injure yourself. Remember, you must warm up your muscles and loosen your joints before you use them. You need to increase your body temperature and circulation before you can safely stretch. A warm and relaxing bath is the perfect environment in which to prepare the body for activity.

To sum up, we need flexibility both of body and mind. The added rewards you'll get from combining yoga, stretching, breathing, and meditation will result in extended vitality. You will feel freer to reach out and catch the best pleasures and satisfactions life has to offer.

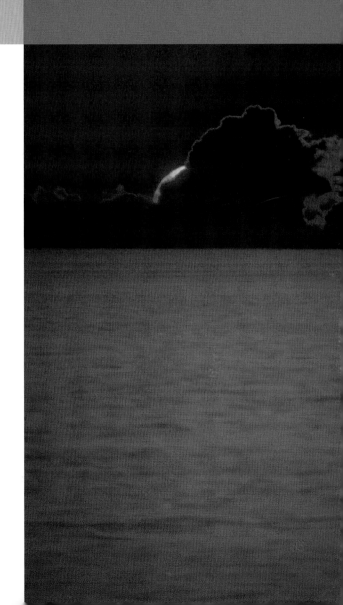

Conclusion

About the Authors

Marjorie Jaffe, a lifelong fitness expert, is the president and founder of Back in Shape Exercise Studio in New York City. Marjorie is the creator and director of the In Home Spa and Back in Shape Travelling Spa Vacations. She is the author of two adult exercise books as well as a Reader's Digest Books contributor.

Books by Marjorie Jaffe

The Muscle Memory Method. M. Evans and Company, 1997. Spanish edition, 1999.

Get Your Back in Shape. Simon & Schuster, 1984, 2nd printing 1985. Published in London by Thorsons' Ltd.

Reader's Digest: The Complete Manual of Fitness and Well-Being. Viking, 1989, Contributor and consultant, author of chapters on exercise and fitness.

Reader's Digest: Practical Problem Solver. Viking, 1990. Author of chapters on exercise and fitness.

Barbara Isenberg is the founder of the North American Bear Company, which designs and manufactures gifts and children's toys. Barbara has successfully marketed her products in both the adult collectible market and the children's toy and gift market. She has been a freelance product columnist for *The New York Times* and is the co-author of three children's books.

Books by Barbara Isenberg

The Adventures of Albert the Running Bear. Clarion/Division of Houghton Mifflin, 1982.

Albert Gets the Jitters. Clarion/Division of Houghton Mifflin, 1987.

Barbara and Marjorie co-authored *Albert the Running Bear's Book of Exercise.* Clarion/Division of Houghton Mifflin, 1984.

And soon to be published, a series of Muffy VanderBear—Chronicle/Children's books.

About the Models

Edwige Gilbert has been a friend and colleague of author Marjorie Jaffe for over 15 years. Edwige is the creator of "Nouvelle Yoga" and "Nouvelle Workout," two classes that she offers in New York City and at conferences throughout the United States. She is the founder of New Life Directions, which specializes in fitness/wellness programs for corporations, health clubs, and individuals. Her healing approach employs a wide variety of Eastern and Western techniques that include Yoga, Qi Gong, and hypnotherapy to develop balance between mind, body, and spirit.

Deborah DeVoursney has lived in The Farm Community in Summertown, Tennessee since 1973. She has studied yoga for 14 years and taught for 11 years. She has a studio on The Farm and teaches in the local college as well as various other locations. She has studied with Rodney Yee, Judith Lasater, Doug Keller, J. J. Gormley, Mary Paffard, Barbara Benagh, and other renown yoga teachers. Deborah combines the various yoga styles into an eclectic blend of yoga and pranayama.

Tal Zadok Kazaz is a native of Israel and has been studying yoga since he was 13 years old. He has been training and teaching shiatsu for five years and is also working with acupuncture and Chinese herbal medicine. In addition to his studies, he started a yoga practice for inmates at an Israeli prison, which has continued since he left the country. While visiting in the United States, he has been staying at The Farm in Summertown, Tennessee, where he has been teaching shiatsu.

BOOK PUBLISHING COMPANY

since 1974—books that educate, inspire, and empower

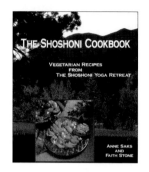

Becoming Vegetarian

Vesanto Melina, R.D., Brenda Davis, R.D., and Victoria Harrison, R.D.

1-57067-013-7 $16.95

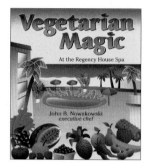

The Shoshoni Cookbook from the Shoshoni Yoga Retreat

Anne Saks and Faith Stone

1-913990-49-3 $14.95

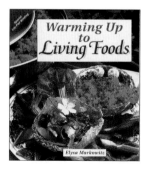

Vegetarian Magic at the Regency House Spa

John B. Nowakowski, Executive Chef

1-57067-100-1 $19.95

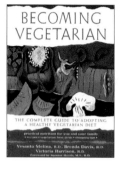

Tofu Cookery

ed. by Louise Hagler

0-913990-76-0 $16.95

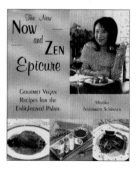

The New Now and Zen Epicure

Miyoko Nishimoto Schinner

1-57067-114-1 $19.95

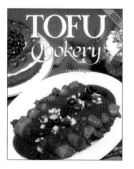

Warming Up to Living Foods

Elysa Markowitz

1-57067-065-X $15.95

Purchase these vegetarian cookbooks and health titles from your local bookstore or natural foods store, or you can buy them directly from:

Book Publishing Company
P.O. Box 99
Summertown, TN 38483
1-800-695-2241

Please include $3.95 per book for shipping and handling.

To find your favorite vegetarian and yoga products online, visit:

www.healthy-eating.com